WEIGHT LOSS

FOR

MATURE WOMEN

HOW TO LOSE WEIGHT AFTER 40 AND GET BACK IN SHAPE FAST

Table of contents

Introduction

Obesity and being overweight are two very serious concerns affecting millions of people all over the world. People have become more materialistic. People now tend to gauge their success in terms of their bank balance. They believe that the more they earn, the more they will be considered successful and as a result they will be respected more in society. In this regard, the media has had a huge part to play.

Whenever we switch on our televisions, we see people enjoying the good life, spending millions in casinos just for the sake of fun, writing blank cheques and enjoying the extravagances in life. And then we see these people being celebrated and idolized. As a result, we tend to measure our lives with the same scale. The United States of America is the country that is most plagued by this problem. In order to earn more, its residents work inhuman hours every day without any regard for sleep, diet or exercise.

When we are younger, our bodies are more energetic and are able to cope with the toughest of conditions with ease. However, when we enter into our midlife, that is, around 40 or 50 years old, the effects of our choices start to kick in. The body, no longer able to withstand the demanding routine, starts to show signs of wear and tear. And the biggest and most dangerous manifestations of an unhealthy lifestyle are obesity and being overweight.

Obesity is the root cause of a lot of health related issues. Mortality rates have gone up considerably ever since there has been an increase in the number of overweight and obese people all over the world. Diabetes, heart attacks, joint pains, sleep apnea, blood pressure, organ failure, kidney problems and so much more. All of these problems are a result of unhealthy lifestyles. According to some medical reports, obesity might also cause certain types of cancer. Hence, it is clear that this is something that clearly needs to be addressed.

If we survey our daily routines and make a list of everything that happens throughout our day we will see where the problem lies. It is quite rare in a competitive country like the United States that people get at least the 7 hours of sleep recommended by experts. Similarly, as people have little or no time to prepare meals for themselves, they tend to go for fast food as it is more convenient and time-saving for them. However, fast foods are a very unbalanced diet which drastically increases your chances of becoming overweight. Furthermore, we can see that many people work 10-12 hours a day. This means that they rarely have any time for exercise and other outlets that are crucial for your physical and mental health. As a result they become lethargic and depressed.

Throughout the course of this book we will look at some of the problems associated with obesity and being overweight, especially in middle aged women. This book is divided into three main chapters. We have already established what the problem is, 'Obesity in middle aged women'. The other topics of discussion in our book will be:

1. The Causes
2. The Symptoms
3. The Solutions

As you can see, we will start off by discussing some of the root causes of being overweight in people. Then we will move on to discuss some of the symptoms that are clear indications of an unhealthy lifestyle. And finally, we will conclude by discussing some easy and effective ways to counteract this problem and live a healthy life.

SECTION I

The Causes

As we shall see throughout the course of this chapter, there are numerous factors that can cause obesity. However the first on our list, as many of you can guess, is dietary imbalance.

Dietary Imbalance

Dietary imbalance, or energy imbalance as it is also known, is a state when the inputs of the body do not equal the outputs. In this case, the inputs refer to the food that we consume daily. Whereas the outputs are the functions that we perform that use up the energy attained by digesting this food. When the food is digested in our alimentary canal, its final state is energy. Energy is required for all the bodily functions. We need energy to breathe and to move. Our heart needs energy to pump blood all over the body.

The food that we eat can also be quantified in the form of energy. If we take a look at the wrapper of a Snickers bar for example, we can see the label says that the bar contains 488 calories. As per scientific definition, 1 calorie stands for:

The energy needed to raise the temperature of 1 gram of water by 1 °C

Everything that we eat has an energy value which amounts to the number of calories contained in it. Having said all that, we can now begin to understand what is meant by an energy imbalance in the body. Dietary imbalance or energy imbalance occurs when we take in more energy (i.e. food) than is required by the body. There is another sort of energy imbalance that occurs if we consume less food than is required for the body, known as malnutrition, however the focus of this book is obesity.

Psychologists have suggested that eating disorders can be linked to the psychological conditions of a person. We have heard the phrase 'stress eating' a number of times. People often start overeating when they are feeling stressed, dejected, grievous, and rejected or any number of afflictions that can have a negative impact on the human mind. Some people have it in their subconscious that they need to eat lots of food every day and often have mood swings if this does not happen.

Eating processed food and fast food like burgers and fried chips is one of the leading causes of obesity amongst children in the United States. Other than that, some people are addicted to bakery products like cakes, pastries, muffins and so on.

Inactive Lifestyle

The choice of our lifestyle has a huge impact on the condition of our body. Nowadays, people have become more lethargic. This is because mankind has found a solution for almost everything that requires physical exertion. For example, before the invention of escalators and lifts, people used to use the plain old staircase to reach their destinations. And in doing so they were indulging in a cardiovascular exercise that helped provide the essential physical exertion required to keep their blood flowing and keep the body in good working condition.

However, now if we are given a choice between a normal staircase and an escalator, most of us would opt for the escalator. People have also become less fond of outdoor activities. This is a problem that plagues the male and female population alike. When we return to our homes after a tiring day's work, we prefer to sit back in our sofas and watch television ra0ther than go outdoors for a walk.

The importance of physical activity needs to be realized if we really are to bring a positive change in our lives. Many middle aged women believe, or want to believe, that they can shed some pounds just by dieting. This is completely untrue and in most cases, there can be no improvements without exercise. Physical exertion is necessary because it puts demands on our cells to provide energy. Cells then utilize the energy sources in our body, which are food and fat deposits etc., to meet the energy demands. Hence we are able to maintain the energy equilibrium in our body. Without any exercise, the excess food in our body is converted to fat which is then stored in the body and contributes to the increase in weight.

Inadequate Sleep

Although our sleeping patterns are somewhat related to our choice of lifestyle (as discussed above) this topic deserves separate mention here because it is somewhat overlooked by most of us.

Sleep is an important natural phenomenon. It is a built in restart system for the mind. It allows the body to perform self-repair and maintenance operations in order to make sure that all the body's functions are performed at the optimum level. Hence, we can easily deduce what would happen if we do not get enough sleep. Depression, memory loss, disruptions in concentration and other such symptoms are all manifestations of sleep deprivation. But perhaps the most concerning symptom is weight gain.

Studies have revealed that women who sleep too little or too much have a high tendency to gain weight as compared to women who sleep between 7-8 hours each night. Middle aged women are more prone to this type of weight gain because their natural metabolism loses some of its potency as the years go by. It is important to note here that 7-8 hours is not the only amount of sleep that is acceptable. It depends on each person. Some people can feel fresh and revitalized with only 6 hours of sleep whereas others might need up to 9 hours of sleep. Thus it is crucial that you understand your bodily needs and adapt yourself accordingly.

In order to further understand how getting the adequate amount of sleep can help us lose weight, we need to discuss two important hormones in the body, ghrelin and leptin. Ghrelin, also known as the 'hunger hormone' is a hormone that is released mainly by the stomach. Its purpose is to instigate the hunger in our body. So whenever we get a craving for food it is the ghrelin hormone which is responsible. When we do not get enough sleep, there is an undue increase in the concentration of the ghrelin hormone in the body. As a result, you will get hunger pangs and will end up eating more food than is required.

Leptin, on the other hand, decreases the food cravings of the body. It also ensures that adequate metabolism rate is maintained so that the energy demands of the body are met. However, when we are not getting enough sleep, the concentration of leptin in our body is decreased. Hence, our metabolism levels go down. So, we can see that if the body is not getting the desired amount of sleep, it will start demanding more food while its metabolism rate goes down. As a result, the energy equilibrium of the body is disturbed and we start to gain weight.

Other Factors

There are several other factors that can contribute to weight gain. From a different perspective, we can also say that all these reasons and those described above are the cause of why many middle aged women find it difficult to lose weight.

For some, the tendency to gain weight is a hereditary condition. It is something that runs in the family. Even after getting the right amount of sleep and exercise, they still end up gaining weight. These people need to exercise extreme caution. Because of their natural tendency to gain weight, such people have to remain vigilant about dietary imbalance.

Other than that, certain medicines and medical conditions like hypothyroidism can also lead to an increase in weight.

SECTION II

The Symptoms

In the previous section we learned about some of the causes that can lead to weight gain in a person. We learned that when the food intake is greater than the amount that is required and digested, the body stores this food in the form of fat. Hence, our weight starts increasing.

Although a bloated belly and limbs are a clear indication of obesity, there are several other symptoms that point towards being overweight. The reason for discussing these symptoms is that people should become aware of what their body is telling them. It might be beneficial for us if we pick up these symptoms at an early stage and perform actions to counteract these problems. Keeping that in mind, let us discuss some of the key symptoms that are common in obese/overweight people.

Type 2 Diabetes

Type 2 Diabetes is one of the major symptoms of obesity. Statistical analyses have revealed that around 80% of the people suffering from type 2 diabetes in the United States are obese. Diabetes is a serious condition and its side effects can really cripple a person's life. People with type 2 diabetes are prone to heart attacks and kidney failures. Obesity can cause the development of gallstones and other urinary tract complications.

Although the exact link between being overweight and having diabetes is not yet clear, there are a number of plausible theories which might explain the correlation. It is suspected that when a person becomes obese, their resistance to the effects of insulin is greatly increased. As a result insulin. the hormone that regulates the concentration of blood sugar level, loses its effectiveness. Hence, the concentration of sugar in the blood rises which ultimately leads to diabetes.

High Blood Pressure

The effective circulation of blood throughout the human body is of vital importance. Blood provides oxygen and other necessary materials to all the organs in order for them to perform their specified tasks. If any part of the body is deprived of blood due to injury or any other complication for too long, that specific part of the body dies and has to be amputated.

The heart pumps blood to the whole body. And the pressure that is applied on the walls of the arteries as a result of the pumped blood is known as blood pressure. Blood pressure is measured in mm Hg (levels of mercury) and it is comprised of two parts: the systolic blood pressure and the diastolic blood pressure. For a normal, healthy person blood pressure should be around 120/80 mm Hg.

However, when our body size increases, so does the amount of cells in the body. This places an increased demand on the body to supply oxygen to all these cells. Hence the heart has to pump harder in order to make sure that the oxygen demands of the body are met. This results in constant high blood pressure. Other than that, the excess fat that accumulates in the body as a result of being overweight can damage the kidneys. Apart from the blood cleansing process, the kidneys also help regulate blood pressure.

High blood pressure can also be the cause of paralysis. When there is too much pressure on the walls of the arteries, there is a chance that the arteries might burst. If this process occurs in the cranial blood vessels, the blood that is leaked from the ruptured walls clots and sticks to that particular part of the brain. This places enormous amounts of stress on the brain and the bodily functions associated with that part shut down. Hence, paralysis occurs.

Sleep Apnea

Sleep apnea is a condition where a person faces breathing problems during sleep. There can be several things that cause sleep apnea. Our sleeping posture, for example, can be a cause. However, sleep apnea is also often associated with obesity.

People who are overweight have fat accumulated in certain parts of the body such as the abdomen, the hips, the arms and legs etc. Fat can also be stored near the neck area. Hence, when such people lie down for the purpose of sleep, the excess fat around the airway starts to constrict the air passage. This constriction causes difficulty in breathing that can be easily recognized by snoring. However, there are other factors as well that can cause snoring which might be related to the nasal cavity.

Because of the stress placed on the air canal by the surrounding fat tissues, inflammation might also occur. Because of this inflammation, overweight people might experience difficulty in breathing throughout the day. This should not be taken lightly as worse cases have resulted in heart failure.

Cancer

Cancer is a terminal disease which is caused by the uncontrolled growth of cells in the body. It can affect many systems of the body such as the brain, colon, blood and etc. Early stages of cancer, if properly diagnosed and treated, can be controlled. However, advanced stages have very high rates of mortality.

Being overweight can lead to cancer. Breast cancer has now become quite prevalent in women especially after menopause. Poor diet and lifestyle can be the cause of cancer. When there is an excess of fat cells in the body, these cells release hormones which alter the chemical makeup of other cells in the body. As a result of these changes, the cells might start to reproduce at an exponential and uncontrollable rate. This eventually leads to cancer.

Obese people are usually fond of fast foods and bakery products. And it is precisely this type of food that can cause cancer. Fast food, also known as junk food, contains high concentrations of sugar, salt and fat. When we drink a fizzy drink for example, there is a sudden influx of these substances in the body. Often the body is not able to cope with this drastic change. As a result the chances of certain types of cancers such as colon cancer are drastically increased.

It is important to note here that apart from being overweight, there are numerous other factors that can increase the chances of cancer. For example, there are some places in Australia where the ozone layer is quite depleted. As a result, the sun's rays in those places are not properly filtered and contain large amounts of x-rays and gamma rays. Exposure to these rays can cause skin cancer. Hence we need to exercise caution.

Other Causes

Apart from the four symptoms that we discussed above, there are many problems associated with weight gain. Such as:

- Heart Diseases
- Osteoarthritis
- Fatty Liver Disease
- Strokes
- Kidney Diseases

Now that we have gone through this chapter, we can clearly see how obesity can lead to severe complications. In order to live a long and healthy life, it is important that we make certain decisions regarding our diet and our lifestyles. Our small efforts in this regard can pay us off in kind in the future.

SECTION III

The Solutions

Coming back to the title of our book, we promised weight loss solutions for older women. There are several challenges faced by older women with regards to weight loss. As we explained earlier, with the passage of time, the e0nergy levels of the body decrease. This has several repercussions. Women during their middle age often find a loss of appetite. This is because the basal metabolism rate decreases. The energy requirements for the body decrease as physical exertions are somewhat limited.

Since we have already established the need to overcome obesity, let us now take a look at some of the techniques that can be employed by older women in order to lose weight and start leading a healthy life again.

Dietary Solutions

To start off we will take a look at some of the dietary solutions that elder women can use in order to effectively lose weight. Most of you would be surprised to know that the best beverage for quickly losing weight is just plain water. Drinking plenty of water every day has a lot of positive effects on the body. It helps us in cleaning out the toxins in our bodies. Whenever we drink water, the alimentary canal is washed out and its motility is maintained. As a result, healthy bowel movements are achieved and food is digested properly.

An important point here is to understand when to drink water. Experts suggest that drinking 2-3 glasses of water after waking up helps in revitalizing and cleansing your body. Another significant measure you can take is to time your intake of water with your meal times. It is highly recommended that you drink water half an hour before your meals. That is the most suitable time and it greatly enhances your digestive system.

Moreover, you can also take limited amounts of water with your meal. This is not as effective as the prior case but it is still acceptable. But once you have had your meal, please refrain from drinking water until about half an hour has passed after eating. We are aware that the stomach contains hydrochloric acid for breaking down food. If you drink water right after a meal, the concentration of the hydrochloric acid is reduced. Hence, the acid does not remain potent enough to completely break down the food.

Vitamin B12 is an important component of the human digestive system. With the passage of time, the body develops a deficiency of this vitamin. B12 plays an important role in converting the fats stored in our body to energy.

Thus in order to lose weight women can ensure that they get adequate amount of Vitamin B12. Food such as eggs, soy milk, fish and almost all the dairy products are good sources of Vitamin B12. However, we must remember that excess of anything is bad. We must maintain a healthy diet plan in order for the effects to really kick in.

There are some substances that older women should try and avoid in order to successfully lose weight. Alcoholic beverages can be quite difficult for the liver to break down and you must remember that your body is not what it used to be. You need to take better care of how much stress you put on your organs and adapt yourself accordingly. Alcoholic beverages such as wine have a high calorie content. And as your physical activity has somewhat lessened of late, it might be a good idea to limit the use of alcoholic beverages.

Leafy vegetables can also help a lot when losing weight. Food such as spinach and kale are excellent options that have low calorie content. Leafy vegetables are an excellent source of dietary fiber. Roughage is extremely important for maintaining healthy bowel movements of the body. These vegetables can be taken in raw form or as smoothies as well. Kale smoothie in particular is known for its revitalizing power. It is a rich source of vitamins and antioxidants which help cleanse the body and regulate the metabolism rate.

Other than that, older women can also increase their intake of broccoli, cabbages, lean meat and boiled potatoes. You must realize that you can no longer run miles on the treadmill or hit the gym with the same intensity as before. Therefore, dietary solutions should be your primary focus and with a proper diet plan, you can start losing weight in no time. However, limited exercise is also crucial and we will now discuss some neat tricks that you can try (along with the proper diet) in order to lose weight quickly.

Exercising Solutions

One thing that must be established here is that exercise is the key to it all. No matter what stage of the life you are in, in order to remain healthy and feel good about yourself you need to exercise. Exercising ensures that the endurance of our body is maintained and that healthy metabolism, blood pressure and heart rate is maintained.

As a middle aged women, you should not be concerned about how hard you exercise. Remember! You should not burden your body anymore that what is necessary. This is because if you exceed the limits of your body, you might end up with an injury. To start off, cardiovascular exercises are an excellent option for losing weight and keeping your heart in a healthy condition. Don't try to do too much all at once. Instead, take your time and let your body acclimate to the change. Walking, jogging and swimming are some excellent cardiovascular exercises that you can try. There are also specialized gyms for this purpose. There you can find trained professionals who have in depth knowledge about weight loss techniques and will get you in shape in not time. You do not need to exercise for long durations. Studies have shown that as little as 30 minutes of exercise each day can greatly help in the weight loss process.

Strength building is also an important aspect of getting back in shape. It will help tone your body so that you start looking good and feeling good again. Strength building exercise will help increase your mobility so that you can feel fresh and energized. It also reduces the chances of arthritis as strength training improves bone density making them stronger and healthier. All that you require is a comfortable bench and a pair of dumbbells. The weight is not that important. Just go with something that you are comfortable with. Normally a 3-4 kg dumbbell will suffice. You can try multiple variants of dumbbell presses and deadlifts to ensure a complete workout of your biceps, triceps, wings, shoulders, chest and back. Other than that, wall pushups and squats are also excellent strength building exercises. Strength building exercises help convert the fat in our bodies into muscle. Hence not only do we lose weight, but we also become stronger.

Flexibility is an important aspect of the human body. Being physically flexible allows you a greater degree of freedom in your movements. Many women over the age of 50 start to shy away from certain activities that they were so fond of in the past. For example, dancing. With the passage of time, as the body becomes more rigid and less forgiving, women tend to give up on dancing because they feel that they cannot move like they used to. However, this can all be resolved with flexibility exercises. Yoga is an excellent option that can help improve the flexibility and balance of the body. Stretching is especially useful for helping out with troublesome hip joints and knees. Not only that, but yoga can also help you to get back in shape quickly making it a very beneficial activity to partake in.

Furthermore, there are balancing exercises such as single limb stance, clock reach, knee marching and staggered stance that you can look into. These exercises along with the proper diet will not only help in bringing down your weight but will also enable you to experience an overall sense of wellbeing.

SECTION IV

The techniques discussed in the previous section gave us a general flavor of what is required if you want to lose weight. However, as this book is focused on weight loss for mature women, we will now take a look at some of the important considerations that are applicable in this case.

Lose Fat Not Weight

For most women, reaching the 40 year mark can be quite a concerning experience. Among other things, women realize that they strength and the energy that they had inside their bodies is slowly fading away. Your choice of actions and lifestyle now begins to manifest their effects which can be clearly observed. First, your look have changed, there are hormonal changes and the menopause as well. Under these circumstances, it is quite possible that women start to lose their will towards betterment. They might feel that there is no longer a need to struggle so much for fitness as they used to before. They let themselves go because they no longer see the incentives that it provides. In such conditions, it is compulsory that you counsel yourself every day and find will and determination to stay in shape.

One thing that needs to be understood here is that your body can no longer afford to lose any muscle mass or bone mass etc. Therefore, you measure of body weight should be different when compared to those who are at a young age. This means that the reading on the weighing scale doesn't necessarily give an accurate description about your weight. Your emphasis should be to cut down on the fat deposits inside the body. Hence, other measurement techniques might be required. For example, the waist size can be one such parameter. Most of the fat at your age is deposited around the waist area. The simplest way to check if you need to lose weight is to see if your waist is more than half of your height. If this is true then you are overweight and you need to do something about it.

Increasing Your Water Intake

As you get older, you might have experienced that your water intake levels have dropped down. This is due to several changes that are happening inside your body. The biggest reason behind this is that your hypothalamus becomes desensitized over the years. Among other things, a critical job of the hypothalamus is to incite the urges of hunger and thirst inside the body. When the hypothalamus becomes desensitized, these urges lose their intensity. Hence, you will end up consuming far less amount of water than which is actually required.

Another reason why mature women often try to avoid the excessive consumption of water can be linked to the dysfunctional urinary system. Many women contract bladder issues and dread the thought of having to go the bathroom every now and then. Thus, mature women may consciously cut down on the use of water as well. But how does low water intake relate to weight gain?

We are aware that for metabolism purposes and for the proper digestion of the food in the digestive tract, water is an essential component. Without water, these processes cannot be performed. Hence, if the water levels inside the body are not what they should be, our body systems malfunction. It is entirely possible that the brain mistakes the body's urge for water with an urge for food. Hence, you might end up feeling hungrier and consume food instead of water which was actually required. Thus, for women beyond the 40 year mark, it is absolutely crucial that they maintain a healthy water intake routine.

Increasing the Protein Intake

One of the major problems faced by women over 40, is that they start losing muscles mass. As we tend to limit the use of our muscles as we get older, the body adjusts itself accordingly. As with any other unwanted substance, the body tries to get rid of the muscle mass which is not used anymore. The muscle mass that is lost in this way is ultimately replaced by fat mass.

The muscle mass and fat mass have stark differences between the two. The muscles burn up a lot of calories every day in order to sustain themselves. On the other hand, fat requires little to no amount of calories. Hence, if you lose your lean muscle, it will become quite difficult for you to lose weight. Another important point to note here is that muscle is a much more dense substance as compared to fat. This means that more amount of muscle can be packed up in a small area. This reveals the mystery of people who look slim yet have healthy weights. Muscle density and fat density can often be quite misleading. People with greater fat mass might weigh the same as people with greater lean muscle mass.

In order to counter the problem of muscle loss, the empty stockpiles need to be refilled. And for that purpose, mature women need to increase their daily protein consumption. Nutritionists believe that for women past the 40 year mark, consuming at least 30g of protein, three times a day is an absolute must. By increasing your protein intake you will instigate a domino effect inside your body. The consumed protein will slowly build your muscle mass. This muscle will burn more calories each day. Hence, in order to meet the energy needs, the metabolism rate of the body will become faster. A high metabolism rate combined with the increased energy consumption will ultimately help you in losing weight by getting rid of the extra fat inside the body.

Having the Right Mindset

There are some beliefs associated with the aging process that aren't necessarily true. For example, many women believe that as they grow old, they are bound to gain weight no matter what they do. It is a part of the natural order of things. Although your tendency to gain weight becomes greater with the passage of time, it is not compulsory that it would be the same case with you as well. Having the right mindset is just as important as the other steps that we have just discussed.

Surrounding yourself with people who have similar ambitions can be quite an uplifting experience. During your weight loss routine, there will be times when you find it difficult to continue. You might not lose weight as fast as you were hoping for and might end up abandoning this cause altogether. Being with your age fellows who have gone through the same will provide a necessary boost to your will and determination. When you see others around you making progress, it will spur you on and enable you to go the extra mile.

Conclusion

Obesity and being overweight are serious problems that have massive ramifications on our lives. Life expectancy and quality of life take a massive hit with uncontrolled weight gain.

In order to lead a healthy and fulfilling life, it is important to strike a balance between the time you devote for work and the time you devote for yourself. Remember that nothing is more important than your health. Even if you have millions of dollars, they are of no use to you if you are not fit enough physically to enjoy your earnings. Therefore remember to take some time out of every day for resting and exercising. Also, be very careful about what you put inside your bodies.

It is never too late to start. All that is required is the will and determination to become better. I am hopeful that you have found this book useful. Weight loss is not at all difficult, even at the latter stages of the life. With the right attitude, diet and exercise, you can start losing weight in no time.